Mudras

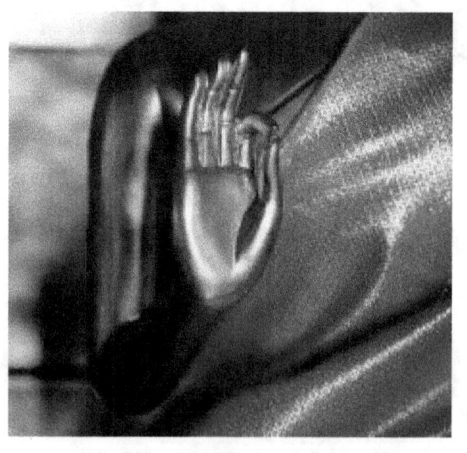

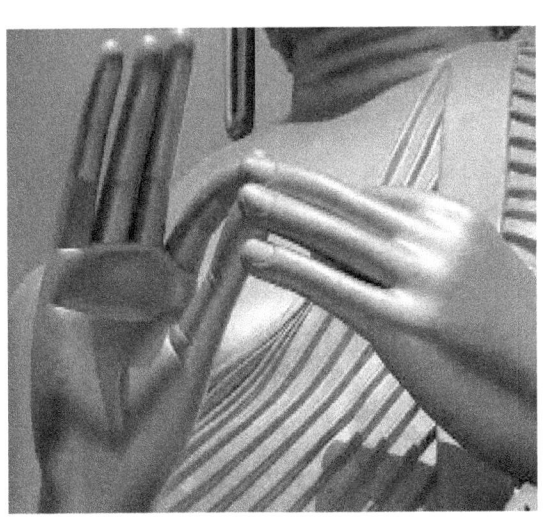

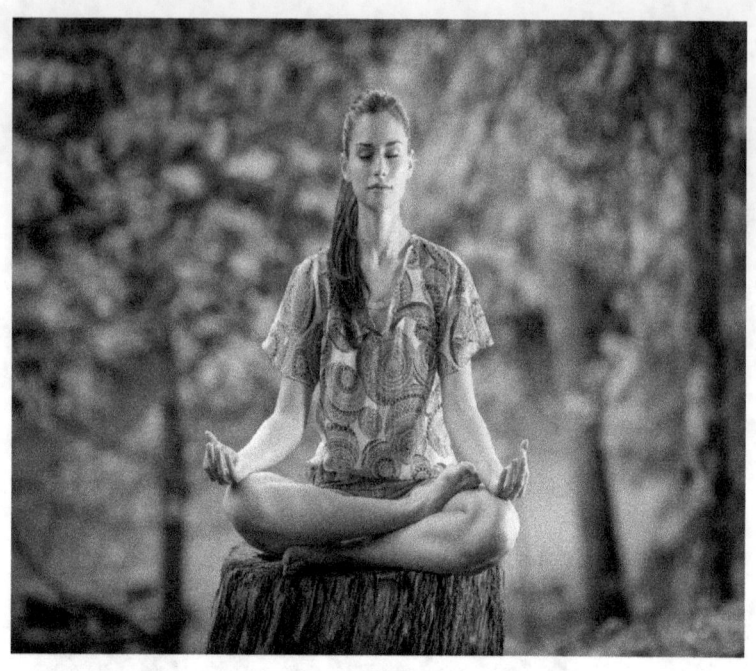

Voice Print

Mudras

*The art of healing &
spiritual growth*

Mudras

Like Yoga, Mudras are a boon to mankind. This science imparts knowledge that leads to self-discovery while providing a means to balance and maintain health independently and maximize the joy of living.

The science of Mudras, a part of Yoga, is based on the fundamental principles of life, namely,

The five elements – akash (ether/space) , vayu (air), Agni (fire), Jal (water) and prithvi (earth).

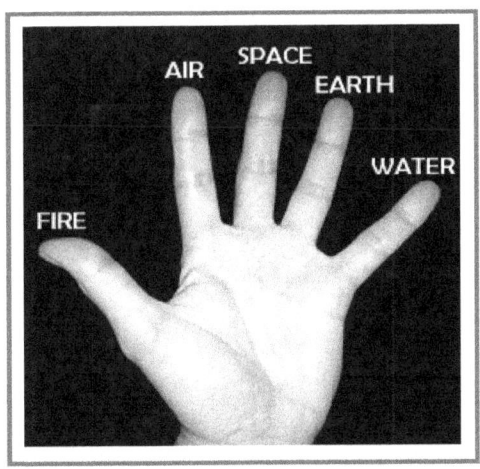

The five pranas –Prana, Udana,
Samana, Apana and Vyana;

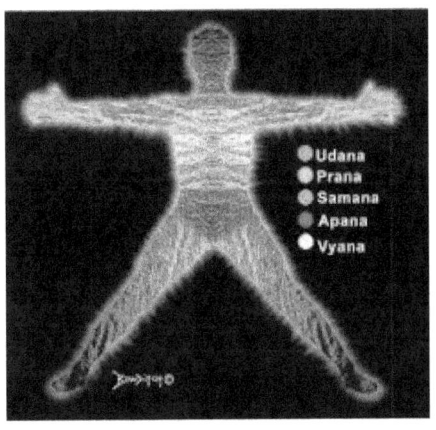

And three doshas – Vata, Kapha, Pitta.

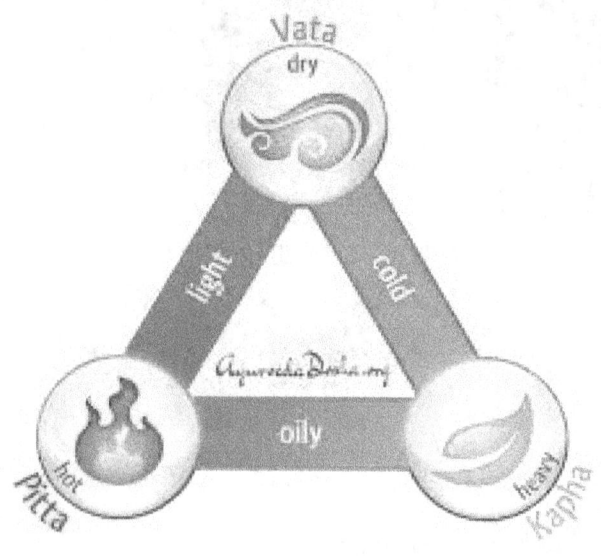

Yogi's and Rishis discovered that the whole universe is composed of five elements mentioned above. They also deduced that the human structure is a miniature from of the universe and hence it's also composed of the same five elements. Therefore they concluded that the secret of god health depends on the balance of the elements within the body and the imbalance in these five elements causes diseases of the body and mind.

Mudras are mainly performed as gestures by fingers, hand positions and also in combination with asanas, Pranayama , Bandha and techniques involving eye movements. Mudras help create and maintain equilibrium in the body elements that results in a healthy life.

The Mudras are comprehensive in nature. They create inner peace and strength, eliminate, fatigue and anxiety, promote physical and emotional health, help relieve stress, depression and anger. They calm the mind, sharpen the intellect and promote, love, happiness, prosperity and longevity.

Originated in India Mudras have lived with us thousands of years through gestures performed during warship and Sandhya Vandana. Various Indian dance forms are also replete with silent eloquence of Mudras. If dance is the language, Mudras are its words.

Some of the original writings on Mudras are found in scriptures like Shiv Samhita, Gherand Samhita and Hathya Yoga Pradipika.

According to the science of Yoga, the attitudes and gestures adopted during Mudra practices establish a direct link between the fice sheaths, seven centres (the Chakras) in the body and the dynamic power Kundalini.

The Five Sheaths:

There is divine spark in us called 'Atma' – the soul and the five concentric layers of matter enveloping the Atma are called sheaths or koshas. The five sheaths are

1. The food sheath – Annamaya Kosha
2. The vital air sheath – Pranamaya Kosha
3. The mental sheath – Manomaya Kosha
4. The intellectual sheath – Vijnanamaya Kosha
5. The bliss sheath – Anandamaya Kosha

The Eight Energy Centres - The Chakras:

The Chakras are energy centres in the spinal column. Each chakra is usually represented as a Lotus. There are seven Chakras in human body that are directly connected with higher centres of the brain.

1. Mooladhara Chakra – It is resides at the base of the spinal column. Its functions are to provide energy, support and balance to the body. This is the seat of Kundalini, the great dynamic power.

2. Swadhishthana Chakra – Spaced two fingers above the Mooladhara chakra is the home of Swadhishthana Chakra. This Chakra is concerned with elimination of waste materials as well as reproductive activity of the body.

3. Manipura Chakra – This Chakra is positioned at the level of navel and corresponds to the solar plexus. It controls the process of digestion, assimilation and maintains body temperature.
4. Anahata Chakra – This Chakra resides behind the base of the heart. It controls the functions of the heart and the lungs and produces virtues like truth, non-violence, love, compassion and forgiveness.
5. Vishuddhi Chakra – Situated at the level of the throat pit it controls the thyroid gland, vocal cords and discriminates the knowledge of the external world.
6. Ajna Chakra – This corresponds to the pineal and pituitary glands lying in the centre of the brain, directly above the spinal

column. This is the command certre, has control over all the functions of human life.

7. Sahasrara Chakra – It is represented by a Lotus having thousands petals and hence the name Sahasrara. It is believed to be situated at the very top of the head. This is the place of culmination of the Kundalini power, the seat of higher awareness and is physically connected with pituitary gland and life system in the body.

8. Bindu Chakra – This is located at the back of the head where Hindus keep the tuft of hair. This is the seat of nectar – Amrit. This nectar is secreted by Bindu Chakra spread throughout the body by Vishuddhi Chakra and the body becomes radiant.

This provides the energy for procreation.

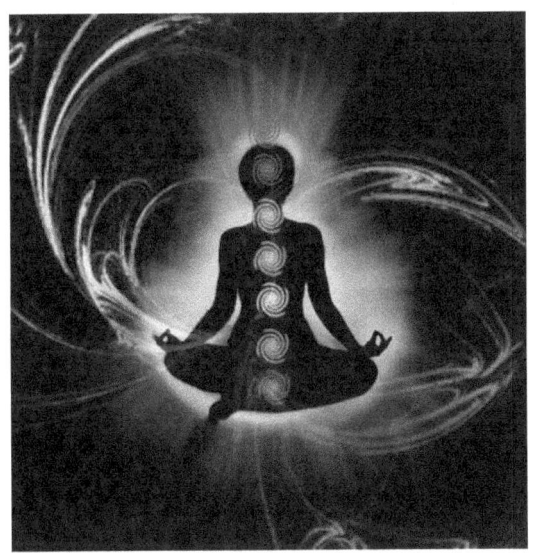

These Chakras are a part of Sushumna Nadi and this subtle body channel is part of the spinal column. On the physical side the spinal column connects the limbs and organs of the body to the brain through a network of channels, the nerves. The Chakras are the junctions.

The brain monitors, coordinates, regulates and controls the functions of the body through these nerves.

Kundalini Power:

Since the dawn of creation the Rishis and Yogis had realized that within the human body there is a potential force that is neither physical, philosophical nor transcendental, but is a dynamic potential force in the material body. This is the greatest discovery of Tantra Yoga.

The seat of Kundalini is a small gland at the base of the spinal cord. With the evolution of natural forces within humans, this gland has reached a point to where it can realize its full potential. In India the entire cultural set up was once organized to facilitate this realization.

When the Kundalini is awakened, a metamorphosis occurs in nature and spirit of the human accompanied by changes in the physical body and the nervous system.

A person with awakened Kundalini power has clarity of vision, a high quality of thinking and a sublime philosophy.

The practice of Mudras affect and influence the five sheaths, the chakras and facilitate the awakening of Kundalini power.

Chanting of Mantras while performing the Mudras would acquire a special aura and the surrounding environment would become lustrous.

According to the science of Mudra, body and mind of human being is governed by the forces of five elements and electromagnetic waves coursing through the channels – the nerves. The disturbance in the five elements cause diseases and imbalance of mind. In order to create and maintain equilibrium in our body and mind we need to take the help of Mudras.

Life is bundle of miracles. This human body has intrinsic power to heal and to be healthy. It has vitality. It can resist diseases and sustain itself.

Man is the greatest creation of God. Within the human body the hand is one of the most important organs. Our body constantly emits electromagnetic power through nerves from the finger tips, nose, lips, ears and toes. So our fingertips become the torch bearers for the Modern age to maintain health.

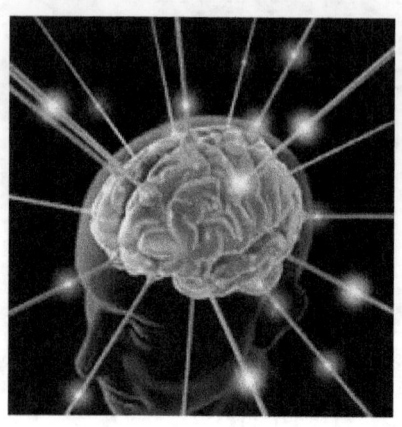

The Brain, Bio-Effect Mechanism & Mudras

A important function of the mind is to instruct the brain to co-ordinate its various neurons to perceive the sensation and then process this perception to affect a proper motor response.

The brain controls the functions of our body via a bi-directional traffic of neurons between itself and the organs. Impulses from organs of sensations are carried by one set of neurons – the Sensory neurons, to the cerebral cortex and the sensory cortex while another set of neurons – the Motor neurons, carry messages from the brain to appropriate organs for action. The two sets of neurons have separate functions. A specific part of the brain, the Thalamus, acts as a relay station in the traffic of neurons. For example – a fly sitting on leg sensation is driven away immediately by swapping of hand, withdrawal of leg, body movement and cognition of incidence. There is immense co-ordination of muscles which brain alone does without loss of time.

Nervous System

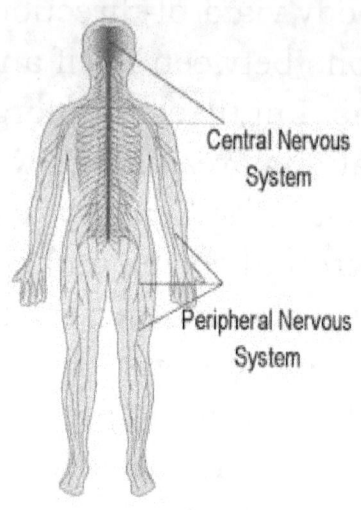

Central Nervous System

Peripheral Nervous System

According to Tantra Yoga Mudras act as a remote control to maintain balance of the five elements within the human body. As we breathe while performing Mudras – fresh air reaches specific parts of our lungs. Mudras enable the brain to activate certain nerve centres and channels in the breathing system to direct the flow of fresh air to specific parts of the lungs. This in turn directs the flow of freshly oxygenated blood to the desired limbs. This is known as the flow of prana – the Vital air.

It is quite incredible that merely by manipulating the fingers we are able to direct the flow of prana to just where we want. Proper breathing them in combination with this specific breathing pattern ensures maximum benefits to the practitioner.

This breathing pattern is as follows:

- Breathe in deep and slow and uniformly for a count of five seconds
- Hold the breath for two seconds
- Exhale slowly and uniformly
- Hold out for a second.

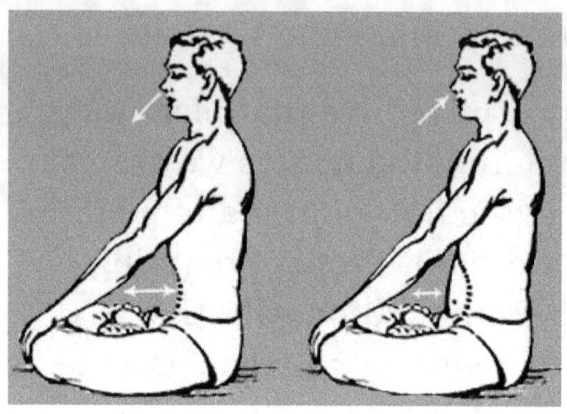

When we perform a Mudra the energy that is being emitted out of our fingertips is arrested and redirected to certain parts of the brain centres from where the proper breathing directs it to parts of the body as per the Mudra.

This is scientific basis of Mudra.

Experiment:

While performing any Mudra combining the fingertip with the thumb tip, the subtle sensation of vibration is felt. Similarly, when we perform Namaste, joining both hands, or place one palm upon the other as in Dhyan Mudra, we feel a strong sensation of vibration. This proves presence of the Electro Magnetic power flowing in our body.

Namaste

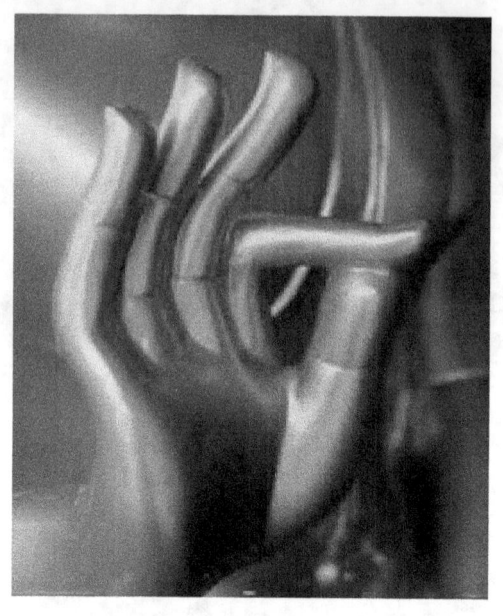

Types of Mudras:

As Mudras are a part of Yoga, they are called Yoga Mudras.

There are five types of Yoga Mudras:

- *Hasta Mudras*: These are the Mudras that are performed by simple finger gestures. So they are called Hasta Mudras. Hasta

Mudra and Mana Mudras, from a relatively large proportion in the universe of Mudras. This reflects the fact from these area of the human body occupies 50% of the cerebral cortex. There are two kinds of Hasta Mudras:

1. Health Mudras
2. Spiritual Mudras

Health Mudras are primarily beneficial in developing and maintaining health. They also have therapeutic usage.

Some of the important Mudras in developing and maintaining health are: Jnana, Prithvi, Akash, Varun, Apan and Pran. Some Mudras used in therapy are: Vayu, Apaan, Vayu, Shoonya, Soorya, Jalodar Nashak and Linga.

Spiritual Mudras are used in worship and meditation. Some of the important Spiritual Mudras are: Namaste, Shankh and Dhyana.

- *Mana Mudras*: These are related to the head and are called meditative Mudras. They utilize the eyes, ears, nose, tongue and lips. Shambhavi and Khechari Mudras are examples of Mana Mudra.

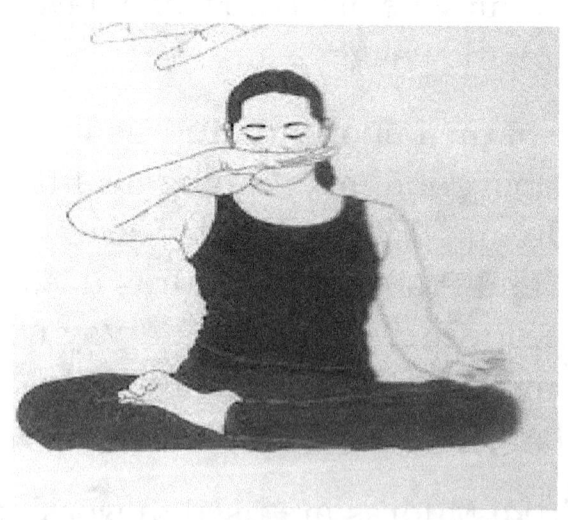

Shambhavi Mudra

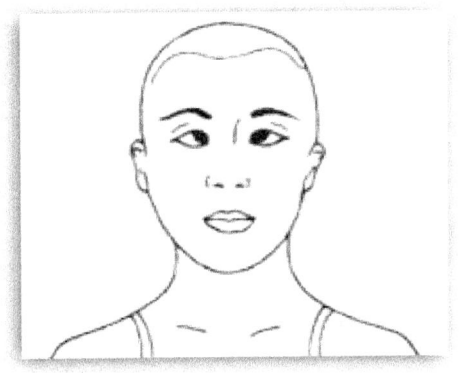

It is said in Hatha Yoga Pradeepika that – *He who succeeds in Khechari Mudra escapes disease, death, fatigue, hunger, thirst and stupor. He who attains this, lives for 100% years.*

Khechari Mudra is performed by reversing the tongue at the throat pit.

- ***Kaya Mudras:*** These are postural Mudras that combine

physical postures breathing and concentration.

- **_Bandha Mudra:_** These are lock Mudras that help in awakening the Kundalini power.

- **_Aadhara Mudras:_** These Mudras redirect Prana from the lower centres like mooladhara and swadhistana chakaras to the brain. These Mudras sublimate the reproductive energy.

Each of these Mudras set up a different link between energy centres and has a correspondingly different effect on the body, mind and Prana.

Significance of Mudras

Through perseverance in meditation and contemplation, the Yogis and Rishis made innumerable discoveries. They could awaken Kundalini power and acquired vitality. They also achieved clairvoyance, clairaudience and telepathy. They perceived their cosmic sound, formed thirty three alphabets of Sanskrit language and realized the vibrations in the body. Accordingly they composed Mantras and Mudras for physical, mental and spiritual well being.

Nature was their laboratory. They realized that there are innumerable species in nature but among them the man is unique in many aspects. He can think, express his ideas, can rediscover the higher planes of spirit hidden within him. The discriminative faculty – the intellect is the rarest gift of nature to man.

Functions of the basic five elements in the human body:

1. Space   -   Akash
2. Air   -   Vayu
3. Fire   -   Agni
4. Water   -   Jal
5. Earth   -   Prithvi

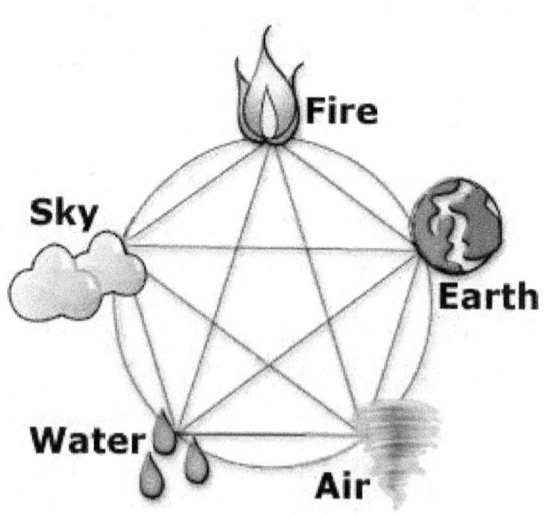

- Akash (Space)- This is an inactive element that manifests itself in that body cavities like the cranial cavity, the paranasal sinuses, the ear cavity, the buccal cavity, the thoracic cavity and the abdomen-pelvic as also the spaces within tubular, bag like organs. Akash creates room within the body, so that rest of the elements can act.
  Akash is associated with sound and therefore hearing. Ear ailments are relieved by the manipulation of Akash element.
- Vayu (Air) – This is the element of movement. All movements of the body and within the body, voluntary as well as involuntary are effected by air. Air is also responsible for our thoughts and emotions and for the movement of the electrical

impulses along sensory and motor nerves. Air is related to the sense of touch and therefore to the skin. Disorder of movements in paralysis or Parkinson disease can be helped by the manipulation of air element.

- Agni (Fire) – This element is responsible for the body temperature and metabolism.

  Fire works on the alimentary system causing thirst, hunger, digestion of food, assimilation of digested food.

  Fire is associated with vision therefore eyes. Disorders like loss of appetite, indigestion and obesity can be helped by the reinforcement of the fire element.

- Jal (Water) – This element is the constituent of protoplasm, blood tears, saliva, digestive juices, sweat, urine, semen, cerebro spinal fluid and fat.

Water is related to the taste and therefore the tongue. Without water the tongue cannot recognise various tastes.

Disorder of water metabolism like dehydration or water retention can be helped by helped by manipulating the water element.

- Prithvi (Earth) – This element is the constituent of body mass, skin, hair, nails, bones, cartilages, muscles etc.

  An excess of earth element causes obesity, while a deficiency causes emaciation.

  Earth (Prithvi) is associated with the smell and therefore the nose.

Disorders like leanness, prostration and low immunity can be helped by the manipulation of the earth element.

Good health is the natural consequence of the balance and controlled functioning of each of these five element.

Mudras help to manifest balance in these elements and help to regain health.

All matter including the human body is made up of atoms and atoms are made up of smaller particles. The three main particles making up an atom are the proton, the neutron and the electron. When electrons move between the atoms, a current or electricity is created. Within the human body this electricity is called bioelectricity. This electricity flows in channels called nerves.

The brain is like a ball floating in a fluid called cerebro spinal fluid. It communicates with various parts of the body via the bioelectricity flowing through the nerves.

The Pranic Body:

Prana is life force. According to Yoga physiology Pranamayas Kosha or sheath is made up of five major Pranas which are collectively known as Pancha Pranas. They are Prana, Udana, Samana, Apana and Vyana. Pranamaya kosha governs the area between the Larynx and the top of the Diaphragm.

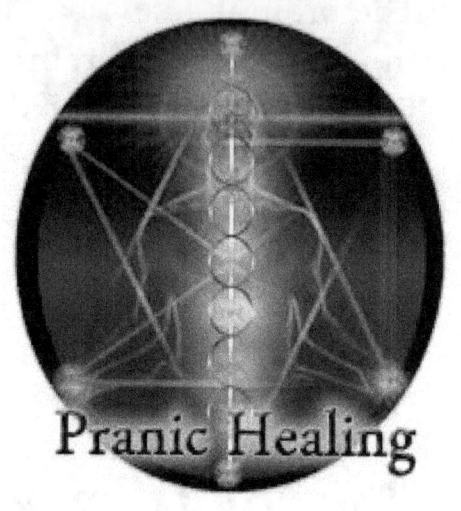

Pranic Healing

All Comprehensive Mudras

- Mudras try to achieve harmony at individual level and universal level.

- Mudras have very extra ordinary powers. The practice of Mudras brings about a quick and fundamental reversion of destructive changes in the human body. They develop virtuous, socially amicable, nonviolent, pious and courteous disposition.

- Mudras are universal in application. They will benefit all who practice them.

- There are numerous Mudras that are performed during worship, Yogasanas and Bandhas.

- The science of Mudras is very exact and perfect.

- Like the universe our body is composed of five elements. A balance among these five elements establishes good health while an imbalance causes disease.

- By the practice of Mudras an element in the body can be increased/decreased to bring it to an optimal level. The optimal level of the element in the body indicates health and happiness. Excess or deficiency of the element induces sickness. Specifically the practice of Mudras can bring about substantial change in the tendons, arteries and glands.

- Mudras are like yogic injection and yogic tranquiliser. Some of the Mudras can balance an element within the body in 45 minutes or less, whereas some other Mudras have an immediate effect. Practising Mudras regularly can cure sleeplessness, arthritis, memory loss, heart problems, impaired hearing, grey hair, incurable infections, blood pressure, diabetes, congested chest and many more ailments.

- Mudras add to facial beauty. In the case of some Mudras, performing them with the right hand, have a positive affect on the left side and vice versa. For example, there is only one artery that supplies pure blood to both side of the body. When we perform Vayu Mudra with the right hand, the flow of blood within this artery gets redirected to the left side thus helping reduce the pain in the knee joint of the left side.
Life is beautiful and one needs the proper attitude to realize it. Mudras like the Gyan Mudras, Prithvi Mudra and Prana Mudra help in building a positive attitude.

Knowledge of Mudras can prove to be of immense help in the progress and protection of the entire human race.

Mudras in the Present context:

- Mudras are an excellent alternative therapy.
- Mudras are not only therapeutic but also prevent ailments, They are very effective.
- Modern medicines can be double edged swords. They have an immediate impact but can have side effects too. They are very expensive, whereas Mudras therapy is cost free.
- Mudras are natural, simple and gentle. They are miraculours.
- Though Mudra is a delicate therapy, we can regain our

health without any difficulty.

- There is no medication in Mudras. Therefore there is no reaction of chemicals.
- There are no ultra sophisticated instruments involved. We need not depend on anybody for treatment.
- Mudras being universal they can be performed anywhere and any time and by anybody.
- Mudras cure all kind of illnesses simple or serious.
- By performing Mudras one can utilize time profitably and can attain radiant health.
- Mudras even help semi conscious or unconscious people. Rubber bands can be used to maintain

thumbs and fingers in specific positions.

- Many doctors and researchers have approved Mudras and they have faith in this technique.

The origin of the Universe and the great five elements

Nature is hte original cause of the universe. There are three quilities in the creation and they are called, the three Gunas.

1. Satwa – Leads to Knowledge and happiness
2. Rajas _ Leads to action for fulfilling desires
3. Tama _ Ignorance and lethargy

These three gunas get disturbed and they continuously transform into another.

Mudras and health dimension:

Mudras assume a new dimension as they help humans to sustain health naturally like other species. Hasta Mudras are formed with fingers. The five fingers of each hand represent the five elements of the body.

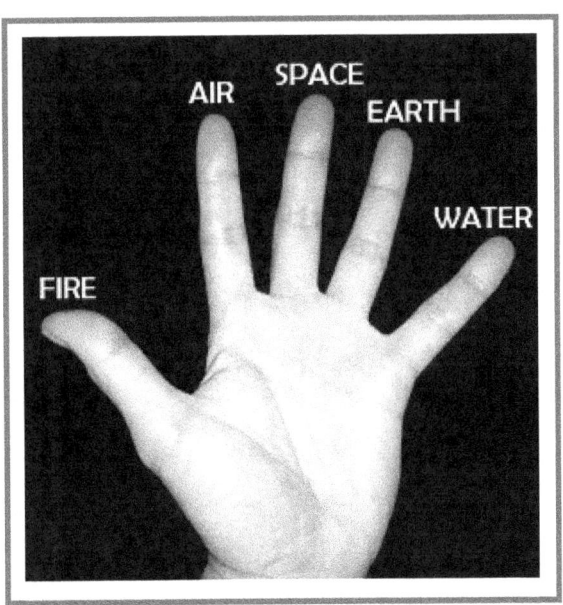

**Finger
Element**

Finger	Element
Thumb (Fire)	Agni
Index finger	Vayu (Wind)
Middle finger (Space)	Akash
Ring finger	Prithvi
Little finger (water)	Jal

Agni is supreme among all the five elements as it is able to control the other four elements.

Similarly the Thumb is the most important among the five finger of the hand. Thumb support the other fingers to function as we desire. Therefore thumb is called Agni. Thumb is responsible for balancing, decreasing or increasing the other elements by forming Mudras. We can manipulate fingers and thumbs in various gestures and regulate the element, thereby restoring health.

Guidelines for Mudra Therapy:

1. Balance, decrease and increase

- Touching the tip of the figure and thumb balance the element represented by the finger.
- Touching the finger tip at the base of the thumb decrease element.
- Touching the thumb tip to the base of the finger increases the element.

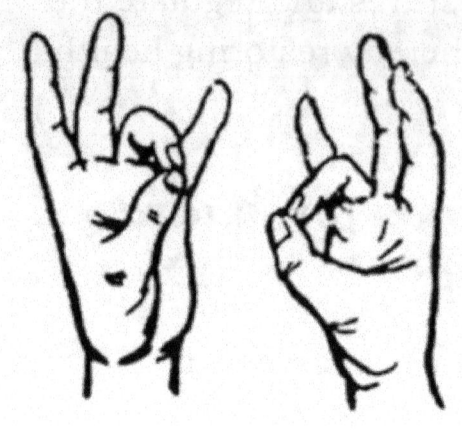

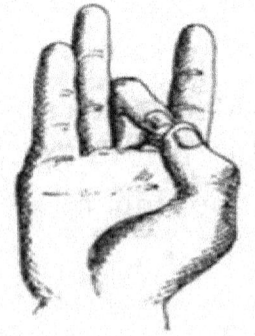

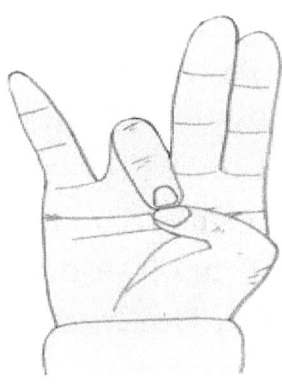

2. A light contact between the tips of the thumbs and the fingers is sufficient. One need not apply pressure.

3. Fingers not actively involved in the Mudra should be comfortable straight.

4. Whenever possible perform the Mudra with both the hands. Perform Mudra with one hand when there is problem in the opposite side.

5. Mudras can be practised anytime, anywhere, while sitting, standing, walking,

travelling, watching TV, listening to music.

6. Mudras can be performed by anybody and facing any direction. Mudras are Universal.

7. Chanting of Mudras (e.g Om, Gayatri, Om Namah Shivaya)

8. Even passive performance of Mudras using rubber bands, sticking tapes for unconscious/insane people or for children while they are sleeping, proves beneficial.

9. Mudra Therapy can be combined with medicines or Yoga therapy. Previously prescribed medication may be continued till well being is established by the doctor.

10.   For general well being, six Mudras are to be practiced everyday for ten minutes each,

They are – Jnana, Prithvi, Apan, Pran, Vayu and Dhyan.

During therapy the specific Mudra is to be practiced for 50 minutes followed by Pran Mudra. If there is time constraint, the 50 minutes practice may be divided into three smaller practices consisting of 15 minutes of practice of the specific Mudra followed by 5 minutes of Pran Mudra.

Some Mudras show their effects immediately. e.g Shoonya Mudra cures vertigo within a few seconds. Similarly, Apan Vayu Mudra gives instant relief during a heart attack. In case of chronic diseases Mudras like Vayu, Soorya and Jalodar Nashak can show their effect within eight to fifteen days.

11. Mudras have capacity to withdraw addiction – e.g Smack, LSD, intoxication and other mental maladies. Regular practice of Mudra can control bad habits like lying and thieving.

12. Pran, Apan, Prithvi and Jnan Mudra can be practised for an unlimited time. Other Mudras must be practised till the illness persists.

13. Healthy people regularly practicethe above four Mudras, so that they would remain healthy throughout their lives.

14. While performing Mudras, placing the hands on the thighs/ knees creates another pranic circuit that stimulates the gupta nadi – hidden channels in the thighs and helps stimulate the energies at Mooladhara Chakra. This

results in increasing energy within the body.

Classification of Mudras:

Developmental Mudras –

Some Mudras are practiced to develop and maintain radiant health. These Mudras can also be performed by ailing people to regain health. They balance the elements and help us to be evey healthy. They are to be practised for 10 minutes every day.

Examples of such Mudras are:

1. Janna Mudra: Performed to increase brain power, improve memory, attaining peace and to remove tension.

2. Prithvi Mudra: Performed to attain balanced health of 5 sense organs, good blood circulation and for energy.
3. Apan Mudra: For good digestion, for healthy gums and teeth, for healthy excretory system, for elimination of wastes and for immunity.
4. Dhyan Mudra: For peace of mind.
5. Pran Mudra: For removal of fatigue, for provision of vitamins, for immunity, for stamina and vigour, for maintaining health of eyes, for helping other Mudras to be effective.
6. Vayu Mudra: Everyday after meals to prevent flatulence, gas problem.

Jnana Mudra

Jnana Mudra is also known as Mudra of Wisdom. Jnana Mudra balances Vayu in our body and steadies the mind.

Jnana Mudra also known as Gyan Mudra

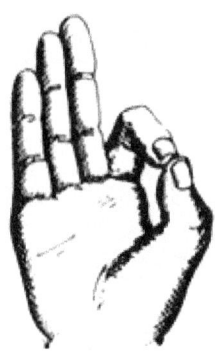

Formation: this Mudra is formed by joining together the tips of the thumb and the index finger.

Effect: Vayu causes movements and thoughts. Agni is related to the brain. When the tips of the index finger and the thumb join together the Vayu gets stabilized. Vayu and Agni together control the mind. That is why this Mudra is called Jnana Mudra – Mudra of *WISDOM*.

 At the top of the thumb lie the points of the endocrine glands Pituitary and Pineal. Performing this Mudra balances their secretion.

In modern times stress / tension / worry / fear have increased and these often disturb all endocrine glands.

Therefore balancing these glands with Gyan Mudra becomes very crucial.

Benefits:

- Tendons, veins become strong.
- Mental power of grasping, concentration and memory increases.
- Empower the mind causing a positive effect on emotions and leading to enlightenment.

- Facilitates movements of electrical impulses along nerves.
- Empowers the Pituitary gland and thereby the entire system of endocrine glands.
- Empowers the muscles both voluntary and involuntary.
- Disorders of the nervous system like cerebral palsy, alzheimers disease neuritis are rectified.
- Degeneration of the retina and optic atrophy are set right.
- Bad habits like addiction, intoxication can be overcome.
- Violent and crul behaviour is due to mental imbalance which would be overcome by this therapy – jnana Mudra 50 minutes followed by Prana Mudra 15 minutes..
- For students Jnana Mudra is a boon. This improves memory, development concentration and

improves brain power. Mental development is manifold.

- Mentally retarded children will benefit – when they sleep, put a band around the Jnana Mudra as there is no time limit to perform this Mudra.
- Tension is removed, anger is pacified.
- Soothes irritability, harsh behaviour.
- Aids in withdrawal from Smack, LSD, Morphine, Bhang, Charas, Cocaine and Ganja.
- Increases commitment to work and selfless devotion to duty.

Akash Mudra:

Space within the body is a part of outer space. A person becomes very broad minded when it is balanced.

Formation: Formed by joining together the tips of the thumb and the middle finger.

Effect: This is a detoxifying Mudra that helps in increasing the space within the body and help elimination of metabolic waste. Negative emotions like anger, fear and sorrow are replaced by positive emotions.

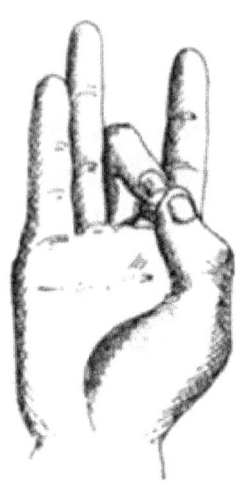

Benefits:

- Helps to detoxify the body by the elimination of metabolic wastes through air, sweat, urine and stool.
- Helps to over come feeling of fullness, heaviness in the body.
- Help to overcome discomfort caused by over eating.
- Helps to relieve congestion and pain in the head due to migraine or sinusitis, ears due to infection, chest congestion, infection, asthma etc.
- Relieves pain in angina pectoris, regularises heart beats and high blood pressure. Practice this Mudra daily for 50 minutes.
- This Mudra is beneficial for any bone related diseases, as the calcium content within the body increases.
- This Mudra is more beneficial at dawn.

Prithvi Mudra

The element Prithvi – earth, is a vital component of bodily tissues like bones, cartilage, skin, hair, nails, muscles, tendons and internal organs. This element builds and invigorates the tissues and increases vitality, strength and endurance. This element is associated with smell and hence it helps to overcome nasal disorders. Prithvi also reduces fire, so an overactive Agni can be pacified.

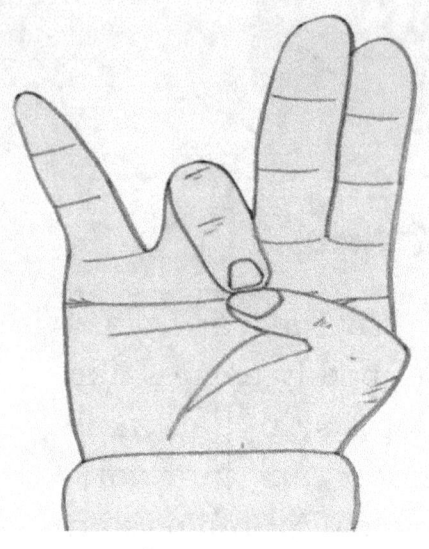

Formation: Join the tip of the ring finger with the tip of the thumb.

Effect: Since the element fire and earth have qualities opposed to earth other, Prithvi Mudra when formed cools the body and reduces the fire and helps overcome disorders of emaciation, fever and inflammation.

Benefits:

- Chronic fatigue, general debility and convalescence can be overcome.
- Treats lacks of stamina or endurance.
- Treats emaciation and weight loss.
- Osteoporosis, Osteo malacia – diminished bone density and rickets can be cured.
- Helps to expedite the union of bones in case of fracture.
- Helps to strengthen the limbs in Polio myelitis, paralysis.
- Dry, cracked, burning skin is pacified.
- Cures skin rashes and urticaria.
- Brittle nails are set right.
- This Mudra provides A,B,C,D,E,K vitamins.
- This Mudra makes one feel happy and contented.

Varun Mudra

Almost 70% of the body is water. Varun Mudra keeps the water balance in the body.

Formation: Join the tips of the small finger with the tip of the thumb.

Effects: Varun Mudra affects the water metabolism. It help to rehydrate cells, tissues, muscles, skin, joints, cartilage etc. The element water, is associated with taste. This Mudra is useful in overcoming disorder like loss of taste sense and dryness of mouth.

Benefits:

- Dryness of the eyes.
- Dryness of the digestive tract.
- Dry cough.
- Dryness of the skin leading to cracks, dry eczema, psoriasis.
- Degeneration of joint cartilage.

- Osteo arthritis.
- Anaemia and cramps
- Deficiency of harmones.
- Scanty urination.

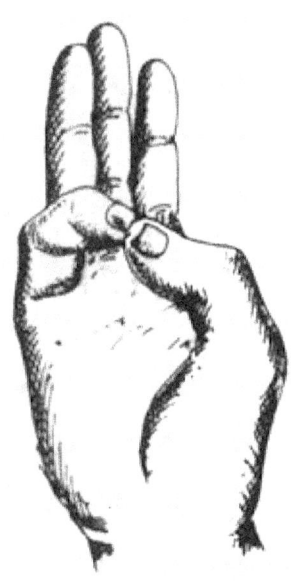

- Loss of taste, tongue disorder.
- Burns.
- Pimples, Itching and all skin diseases.
- This Mudra helps in removing dryness from the body and adds

tenderness, glow and beauty to the skin.

- It is beneficial in removing impurities present in the blood.
- This Mudra preserves youthfulness.
- Unconsciousness due to sunstroke, accidents or over crowdedness can be cured by rubbing the tips of the thumbs and the tips of little fingers.

Vyan Mudra

The current of air – Vyan Vyan, in the vuins is said to be the circulator of the blood in the body. When this air current starts moving very fast in the lungs, arteries and veins the disease is called the high blood pressure. Performing Vyan Mudra 2-3 times a day for 50 minutes each followed by

Pran Mudra for 15 minutes each followed by Pran Mudra for 15 minutes helps in regulating blood pressure.

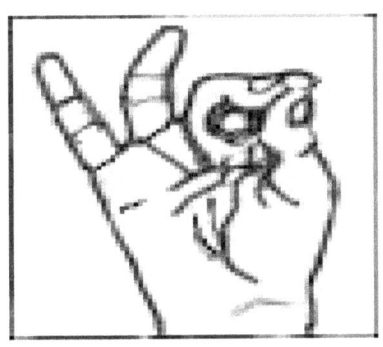

Formation: The tips of Index finger and middle fingers to be joined with the tip of the thumb.

Effect: The speed of the air circulation of Vyan vayu is regulated.

Benefits: Blood pressure either high or low is regulated and balanced.

- Lack of initiative, enthusiasm, slowness of thoughts and perception is corrected with Vyan Mudra.
- Drowsiness, excessive sleep is overcome.
- Intolerance to hert, sunstroke can be averted.
- Excessive sweating, thirst, urination, loose motions and menorrhangia can be overcome.

Apan Mudra

According to yogic physiology, the vital Pranamaya Kosha is made up of Pancha. Pranas – the five winds: Prana, Udana, Samana, Apana and Vyana.

Apana Vayu is concerned with the expulsion of body wastes in the form of sweat, urine, feces etc. Apan Mudra facilitates expulsion of waste from the body and keeps the body clean.

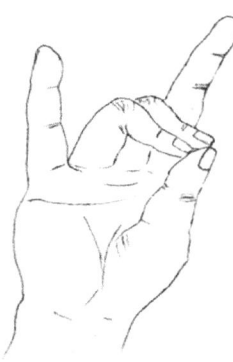

Formation: Tip of the thumb is to be joined to the tips of the middle and the ring fingers.

Effect: Apan Mudra is a combination of Agni, Akash and Prithvi elements.

Combination of these elements improves digestion and provision of calcium and vitamins.

Benefits: ThisMudra helps improve the flow of perspiration, urine and stool. Apan Mudra can be used to overcome the following disorders:

- Anuria – Absence or obstruction of urine.
- Constripation, flatulence, piles.
- Absence of sweet.
- Stomach such as stomach pain, vomiting, hiccups and restlessness.
- Soothes tooth ache. In general, practicing this Mudra everyday for 10 minutes helps maintain healthy teeth.
- Migraine would be cured with Apan Mudra and Jnana Mudra each for half an hour.

Pran Mudra

Pran Vayu is very important Vayu among the ten types of Vayu-s which exist in the body. Pran Vayu is breath itself. It is found in the nostrils, face, heart and respiratory organs. It covers the space till the navel.

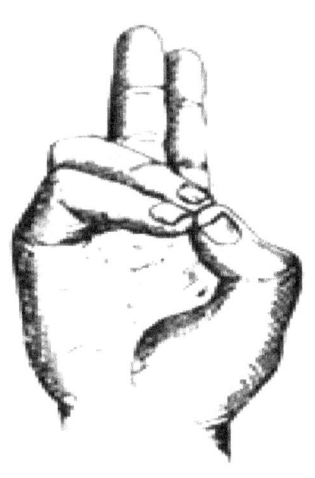

Formation: The tips of little fingers and ring fingers are joined with the tips of the thumbs.

Effects: The major part of our body is Prithvi and Jal (earth & water). Joining the finger tips balancing these elements results in increasing stamina, vitality, strength and immunity. This Mudra starts the flow of vitality, strength and immunity. This Mudras starts the flow of vital energy in our body as if life dynamo has been started. While practising meditation along with this Mudra, the whole body feels the vibration. Practicing this Mudra makes a person mentally and physically strong.

 Benefit: Pran Mudra helps to overcome the flowing disorders.

- Chronic fatigue, debility, low endurance.
- Impaired immunity.

- Mental tension, anger, irritability, jealousy, pride, restlessness.
- Inflammatory disorders.
- Forgetfulness.
- Scanty, burning, urination.
- Burning red, dry eyes, cataracts.
- Dry red hot aging skin, skin rashes, urticaria and leprosy.
- Any ailment of eyes is cured, eyesight is improved.
- Prana Mudra helps remove any kind of deficiency of vitamins A,B,C,D,E,& K. All vitamins are provided by this Mudra.
- Any type of cramps in muscles or veins and pain in the legs are cured.
- Numbness in any part of the body is cured by Pran Mudra.
- During fasts this Mudra can help control hunger and thirst.

Therapeutic Mudras

Vayu Mudra:

When the air element in the body increases because of diet or life style, many kinds of disturbances raise their ugly head. To decrease the Vayu element perform Vayu Mudra and attain balance.

Formation: Index finger tip is to be placed at the base of the thumb and the thumb is to be placed on the back of the index finger gently. Other fingers are to be straight. This is Vayu Mudra.

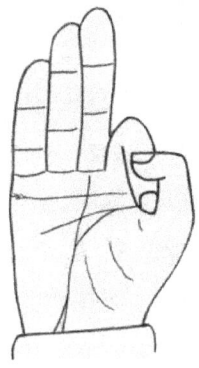

Effect: Excess Vayu is decreased, blood circulation improves and any areas of the body experiencing pain start getting relief.

Benefits: This Mudra acts slowly but steadily. Within 8 to 10 days the results are attained.

- When Vayu in our body accumulates in any part, it causes severe pain and aches. This Mudra can cure such aches.
- The feeling of restlessness or gas formation after meals can be

cured if this Mudra is practised immediately.

- By yawning or by burping the Vayu problem gets resolved.
- Vayu diseases such as parkinsons, sciatica, paralysis, cervical spondylitis and knee pains get cured by this Mudra by regular practice.
- Vayu Mudra helps in balancing the water elements in the cartilage of the joint.
- Gout is cured with continuous practice of Vayu Mudra followed by Pran Mudra.
- Pain in the neck, frozen arm are cured by the Vayu Mudra followed by Pran Mudra.
- Convulsion are cured by regular practice of Vayu Mudra daily for 15 minutes.

Shoonya Mudra

Middle finger of the hand represents Ether-Space-Akash. Space is all over the world and in every cell in the body. The disturbance due to excess Akash element in the body, causes various types of diseases – like cardiac weakness, ear problem, vertigo etc. And Shoonya Mudra helps resolve problems associated with an excess of the Akash element.

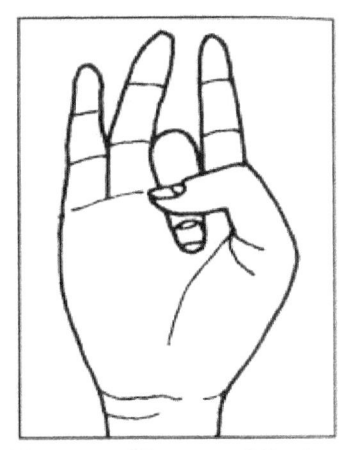

Formation: The tip of the middle finger is to be placed at the base of the thumb and the thumb is to be placed on the back of the middle finger gently.

Effect: The space element is reduced.

Benefit:

- Ear ache subsides immediately.
- Audio weakness is remedied.
- Deafness is cured.
- Dumbness is cured if it is not by birth.
- Numbness in the head, body parts, chest, abdomen can be remedied by this Mudra.
- Ear ailment like pain, tinnitus (noises) acquired deafness will be certainly remedied.
- Severe headache, ear pain, imbalance while walking, pain in the tooth, pain in the throat, pain in the heels, joint pain -

Shoonya and Vayu Mudra to be performed together followed by Pran Mudra.

Surya Mudra

Surya means – the Sun. Surya Mudra generates heat in the body like sun. This Mudra decreases Prithvi element and increases Agni element.

Formation: The tip of the ring finger is to be placed at the base of the thumb and thumb is to be place gently on the back of the ring finger.

Effect: The element Agni is associated with body temperature and metabolism. Practice of Soorya Mudra helps to maintain the body temperature and keeps the metabolism going.

The element Agni is also associated with vision. Hence, this Mudra strengthens eyes and improves vision.

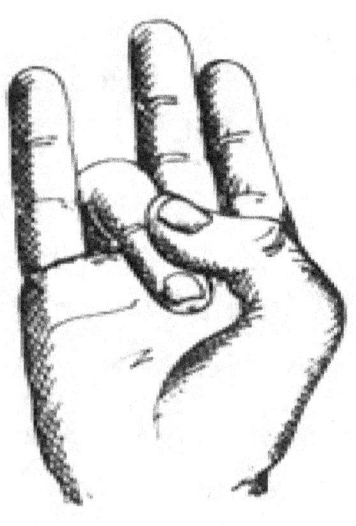

Benefit: Surya Mudra can treat following disorder.

- Abnormally low body temperature,
- Intolerance to cold, shivering.
- Under activity of the thyroid gland causing slow metabolism.
- Obesity, progressive weight gain.
- Loss of appetite, indigestion and constipation.
- Absence of sweating.
- Cold problem like cough, tuberculosis, sinusitis, pleurisy and asthma.
- High cholesterol in the blood.
- Cataract.

This Mudra can be combined with Linga Mudra for better results.

Jalodar Nashak Mudra

Jal means water, Udar means stomach and Nashak means to end. The little finger signifies water element. Jalodar Nashak Mudra controls the excess of water element in the stomach.

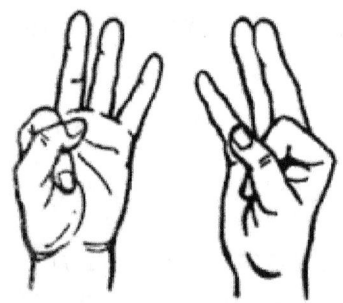

Formation: The tip of the little finger is placed at the base of the thumb and the thumb is placed on the back of the little finger gently.

Effect: Jalodar Nashak Mudra reduces the excess water element in the body, suitably affecting the water metabolism. It can thus overcome water logging within the body.

Benefits: Jalodar is a Sanskrit term for the disease – Dropsy. This disease is caused due to excess of water content in the stomach. This Mudra is named after the curing of the disease – *Jalodar.*

- This Mudra can cure Elephantitis.
- Swelling in any part of the body like face, hands and legs can be cured with this Mudra.
- This Mudra Cures excessive salivation, watery eyes, running nose, hyperacidity, diarrhoea (loose motion)
- Pleusity, effusion in a joint is cured.
- Excessive urination is cured.

Kidney Mudra

This Mudra cures kidney disorders. This has the same qualities like Jalodar Nashak Mudra.

Formation: The little finger and the ring finger tips are to be placed at the base of the thumb and Thumb should be placed over the two fingers.

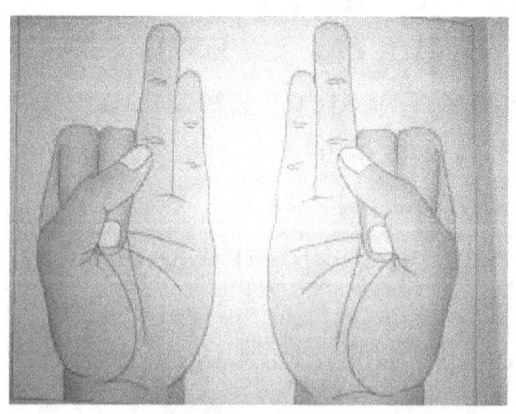

Benefits:

- The problem of running nose is cured.
- Throat pain is pacified immediately.
- Problems of phlegm in the throat and the lungs is cured.
- Helps in curing kidney related problems.
- Helps in curing Dropsy.

Discontinue performing this Mudra when aliment is cured.

Linga Mudra

This Mudra increases bodily heat as it reinforces the fire element.

Formation: Linga Mudra is formed by inter locking the palm but keeping the left thumb erect pointing upwards. This Mudra can be done by reversing the hand too.

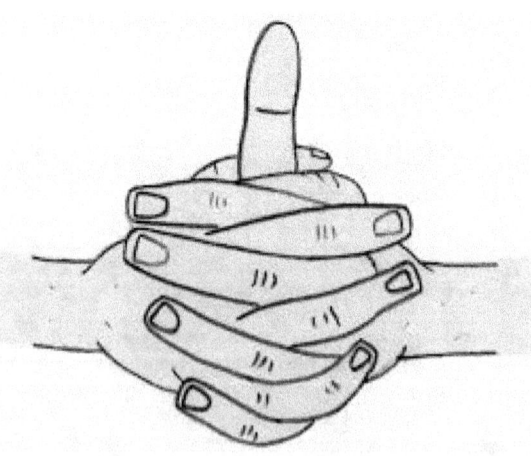

Effect: The fire in the thumb is activated and is able to increase uninhibited.

Benefit:

- Hypothermia – Shivering and chills due to cold weather can be controlled.
- Aliments caused by over production of mucus such as wet cough, colds, sinusitis etc. Can be cured.
- Asthma, bronchitis, T.B., Pleurisy are cured.
- Discomfort experienced in an air conditioned room is relieved by this Mudra.
- Increases digestive powers and also melts excess fat in the body. Give better results when performed together with Soorya Mudra – both 15 minutes each, one after the other.

- Difficulty in breathing can be relieved by this Mudra immediately and one can get good sleep.
- Regulates the flow of the menstrual cycle. Give better results when performed together with Surya Mudra – both 15 minutes each, one after the other.
- When Navel centre is shifted from its original place, comes back to its place by this Mudra.

Special: This Mudra increases heat in the body so this Mudra is to be performed only for 15 minutes or less. Since this Mudra generates heat one much consume a lot of liquids like water, fruit juices, milk, buttermilk etc.

- Any one suffering from acidity, fever and stomach ulcers should not perform this Mudra.

- This Mudra is to be performed only till the problem persists and then it should be discontinued.

Shankha Mudra

In Sanskrit Shankha means Conch.

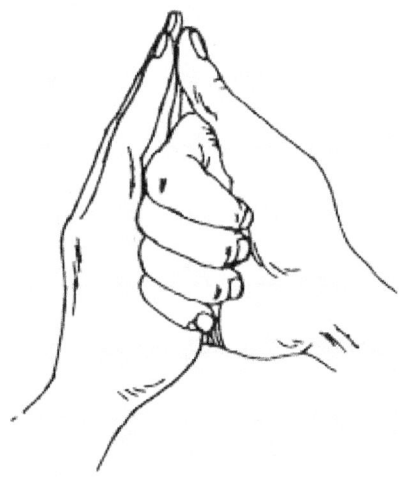

This Mudra resembles the shape of a Conch and hence is called Shankha Mudra.

Formation: Place the thumb of the left hand at the base of the right thumb. This is the point of Thyroid gland in the palm. Fold the fingers of the right hand covering the left thumb. Jointhe index finger of the left hand with the thumb tip of the right hand. The other three fingers of the left hand are to be placed on the back of the right palm.

Effect:

- This Mudra puts pressure on the point of the thyroid gland, thus making it active to remove illinesses related to thyroid gland.
- This Mudra purifies 72,000 nerves connected to the navel centre, there by rejuvenating the whole body.

- This Mudra makes the voice melodious and clean. Removes strain in the voice. Therefore singers, teachers, doctors, lawyers and leaders must perform this Mudra everyday for 10 minutes.
- This Mudra relieves allergies, caused by dust and smoke, so throat becomes clean; also pacifies skin rashes.
- Relieves feverish feeling in the body.
- Relieves burning sensation in the body or body parts.
- Any trouble of stammering, stuttering in speech can be rectified by this Mudra.
- After a paralytic attack, this Mudra helps in dealing with speech problems and speech becomes clear.
- Helps in increasing height of children.

Sahaja Shankha Mudra

This Mudra is a version of Shankha Mudra. Benefits are also the same with a few exceptions.

Formation: Join both hands together interlocking the fingers and press the palms together. Apply a gentle pressure with both the thumbs by laying them parallel to each other on the index finger.

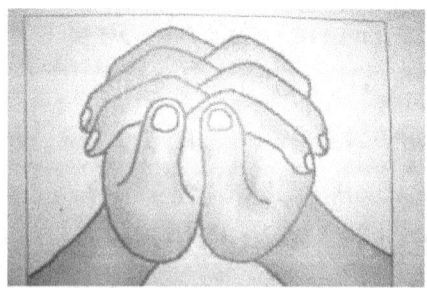

This forms the Sahaja Shankh Mudra.

Effect: According to Yoga physiology, all 10 main nerves get activated and the body becomes very strong with this Mudra.

The ten main nerves are Sushumna, Ida, Pingala, Gandhari, Hasti Jiva, Poosha, Yashaswini, Alamboosha, Kuhoo and Shankhini.

Benefits:

- There is growth in alertness.
- The nerve Shankhini would activate Mooladhara Chakra. The serpent power Kundalini rises towards higher levels.
- Remove the problems associated with the reproductive system.
- Cures piles and problems related to the anus.
- The spinal code becomes straight and gains flexibility.

Aditi Mudra

Formation: Place the tip of the thumb at the base of the ring finger.

Effect: This finger represents Prithvi and the thumb represents Agni, When the Agni touches at the base to the ring finger there is a growth of Prithvi element and also growth of Agni. Therefore there will be weight gain with improvement in stamina.

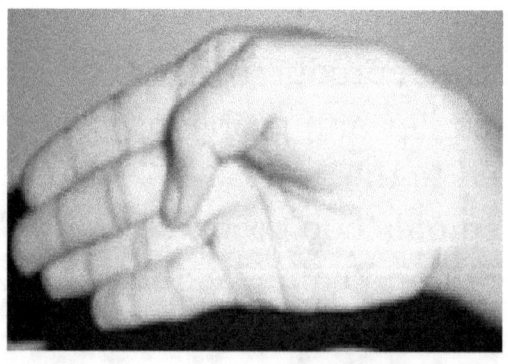

Benefits:

- One can gain weight by a regular practice of 50 minutes followed by Prana Mudra. There will be remarkable weight gain.
- Problem of sneezing continuously in the morning can be cured with the practice of this Mudra Yawning and sneezing during meditation can be prevented by practising this Mudra.

Wish fulfilling Mudra Surabhi Mudra.

Formation: Form Namaste and keep the thumbs apart. Join the tips of index finger and middle finger which are opposite to each other and then join little finger tip with the ring finger tip which are opposite to each other. This is Surabhi Mudra.

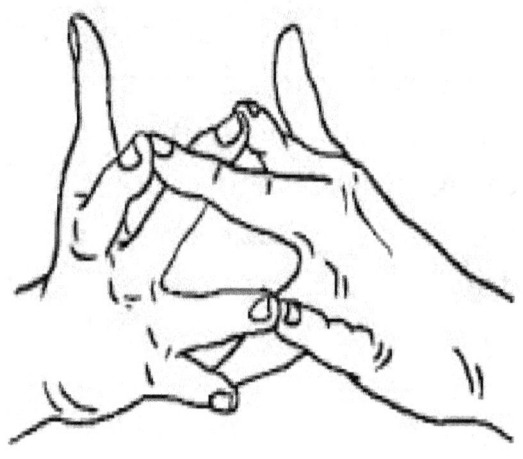

Effect: Thumbs kept apart help reduce the fire. The joining of the tips of middle and index fingers and joining of the tips of ring finger and little finger remove the problems of bile and gout and rheumatism. As the eight fingers come together they activate a number of nerve centres and glands especially Adrenaline, Pituitary and Pineal.

Benefits:

- All the glands Adrenaline, Pituitary, Pineal and Thyroid function better.
- The three Doshas-Kapha, Vata, Pitta get balanced.
- Acidity is cured immediately.
- There is a lot of development in creativily. Novelty increases in every endeavour we take up.
- Desires and dreams are realized.
- To realize our dreams one has to perform this Mudra for 10 minutes every day for at least 15 days.

Hridaya Mudra (Apan Vayu)

This Mudra can save a person from a Heart Attack and hence this Mudra is called the Sanjeevani Mudra, one that gives life to a dying person. This Mudra gives instant result and the pain is reduced immediately.

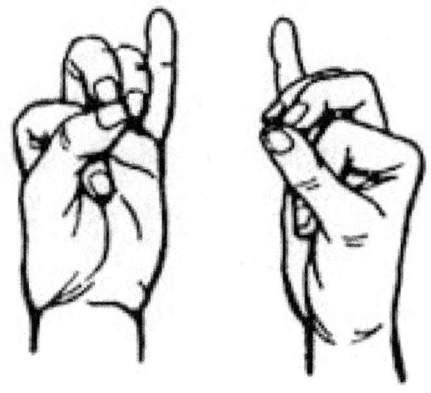

Formation: This is a combination of two Mudras Vayu and Apan. Form Vayu Mudra by placing the tip of index finger at the base of the thumb and then form Apan Mudra by joining the tips of the thumbs with the middle and ring fingers. This can also be formed the other way shown in the picture.

Effect: There is combined effect of Vayu Mudra and Apan Mudra. Vayu Mudra relieves the pain instantly and Apan Mudra maintains space to reinforce blood circulation to the heart.

Benefits:

- When one gets the symptoms of a heart attack this Mudra will act like an injection and helps the person to recover from pain instantly. It reduces excuss gas from the stomach and makes the heart muscles to work efficiently.
- Chest pain, tiredness and perspiration will be reduced immediately.
- This Mudra removes the blocks in the blood veins.
- Cures Constipation.

- Irregular heart beats are regularised.
- Even a little pain in the chest region is pacified by this Mudra. One starts yawning and gives out the excess Vayu from the chest region and one feels comfortable.
- Too much perspiration in the feet and hands is pacified.
- Headaches due to lack of sleep mental worries, over exertion and problems of blood circulations are relieved.
- Beneficial in curing acidity.
- Migraine headache gets relief.
- Beneficial in relieving tooth ache.
- The functional capacity of various organs of the digestive system increases.
- This Mudra cures – Arthritis, Spondylitis, Parkinson and Paralysis.

Yoni Mudra

This Mudra is specially is specially designed for women. The posture of this Mudra is held at the level of abdomen.

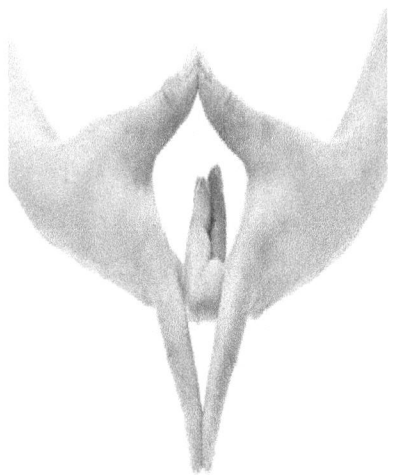

Formation: Join the thumbs and index fingers. Interlock the other finger. The thumb will be facing upwards and the index fingers will be facing downwards.

This can also be performed the other way shown in the picture.

Effect: As the thumbs and index finger touch each other they reflect volume of heat and air waves. Other fingers remain inter-locked would solve the problems of the womb.

Benefits:

- From the age of about thirteen girls have their periods and they get pain in the lower abdomen. Performing this Mudra only for 5-10 minutes relieves the pain.
- Excess bleeding will be regulated

Kundalini Mudra

Kundalini Mudra is associated with the reproductive energy.

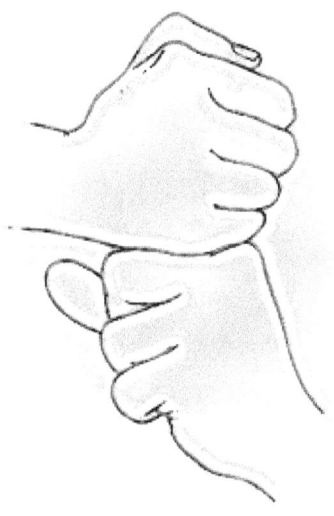

Formation: Form a fist of the left hand and extend the index finger. Cover the index finger with right hand fingers and place the right thumb on the top.

Hold this Mudra in front of the abdomen for 15 minutes, three times a day.

Effect: This Mudra enhances the Kundalini force and the energy is released.

Benefits: This Mudra promotes vigour in the couple.

Pankaj Mudra

Pankaj means lotus. It grows in water and is considered very sacred in India. A number of gods and goddesses like Brahma, Laxmi and Saraswati have lotus are their seat.

We form Pankaj Mudra as a symbol of purity and offering. It is a part of worship.

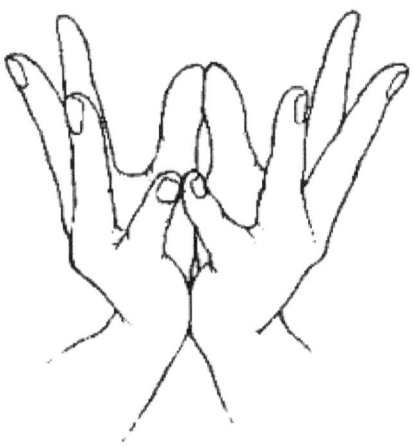

Formation: Join the two palms facing each other. Join the thumbs and the little fingers. From the other finger like a blooming Lotus.

Effect: The Thumbs represent fire and the little finger represent water.

Joining these fingers means purifying the body & mind.

Benefit:

- The mind becomes calm and pure. The body also becomes cool.
- This Mudra pacifies fever in a short time.
- The beauty of the face is enhanced by this Mudra.

Dharana Shakti Mudra

Dharana means to retain the breath for longer time.

Formation: This Mudra has three stages.

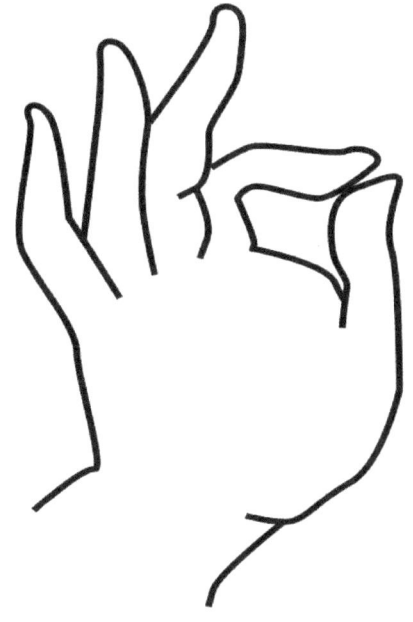

1. Start inhaling with the thumb tips pressing the tip of the index finger.
2. Next press the middle part of the thumb and keep on inhaling for some more time. Retention of breath is still longer.

3. Then press the base part of the thumb and retention of the breath can be still longer.

Effect: The lungs get more oxygen by retention of breath.

Benefit:

- The longer the breath the more is the oxygenation of the body resulting in purer blood and a stronger body. To a large extent, practising this Mudra reduces the total number of breaths in the day. This in turn, increases longevity.

Mushthi Mudra

Mushthi is the tight fist which is the symbol of force.

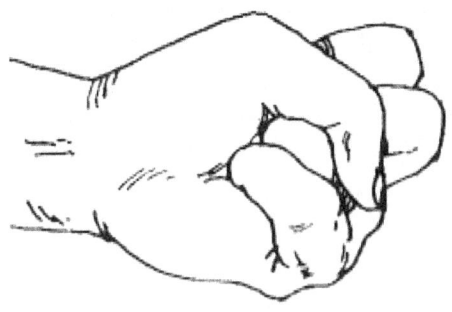

Formation: Form the fist with both hands and place the thumbs on the back of the ring fingers.

Effect: This Mudra is the combination of Vayu Mudra, Soonya Mudra and Jalodar Nashak Mudra which decreases all the four elements there by solving the problems of the excesses of the four elements namely Vayu, Akash, Prithvi and Jal. The Agni affecting Soorya Mudra generates heat and energy in the body.

Benefit:

- When feeling depressed, discouraged or suffering from physical discomforts like: shivering, phlegm in the wind pipe or feeling of lethargy and inertia, perform this Mudra for 50 minutes followed by Pran Mudra.

Namaste – Symbol of Indian Culture

The gesture of Namaste is essentially Indian. It is the symbol of greeting from ancient times. Namaste represents the belief that there is a divine spark within each of us that is located at the heart chakra.

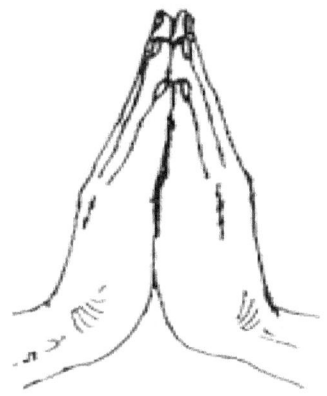

Formation: To perform Namaste we join the hands together and place at the heart Chakra, close the eyes and bend the head.

Namaste also can be done by placing the hands together in front of the third eye between the brows, bowing the head and then bringing the hand down to the heart. This is the deep form of respect.

Effect: Namaste is a Mudra that is rich in flavour, meaning and substance. The Electro magnetic power flowing from one hand to other is felt strongly. One feels strong in body and mind.

Benefit:

- This Mudra frees us from the bonds of ego and makes us humble and pleasant. We feel strong in body and mind as this Mudra removes fear and headache.
- Namaste is uplifting. It gives a sense of gratefulness and waiting to receive blessings of good things to come.

Ashirvad Mudra ---- is blessing Mudra

Youngsters touching the feet of elders with crossed hands is considered very auspicious in India. This is called Namaskar Mudra.

Formation: This Mudra is formed by keeping both palms on the head of the person performing the Namaskar Mudra.

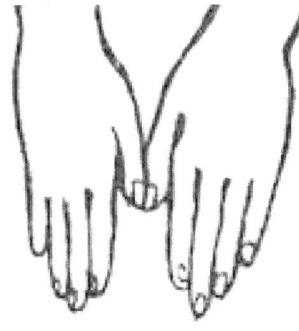

Effect: When the youngsters bow and touch the feet with crossed hands, the blood circulation to their head is increases. When they touch the feet of elders with crossed hands, positive energy and negative energy of both sides get activated.

- During the act of Ashirvad, the positive and negative energy of the two hands touch the hemispheres of the brain as well as the crown Chakra of the person performing the Namaskar. There is a positive and happy feeling that grows in both of them. This way, the Namaskar and the Ashirvad becomes fruitful.

Dhyana Mudra

In Sanskrit Dhyana means meditation. This Mudra is important for one to achieve spiritual progress through meditation.

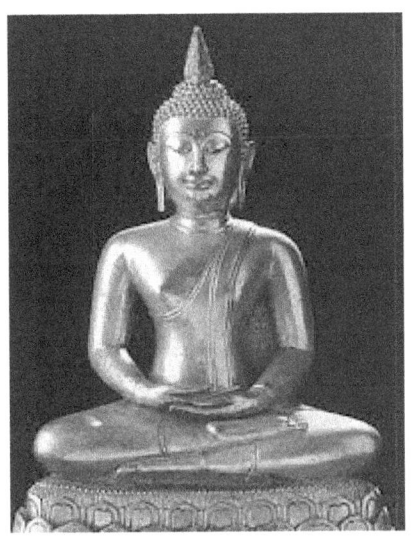

Formation: Being a meditation Mudra one has to assume meditation pose like padmasana, Sukhasana or Siddha Asana. Place the left hand on the right hand with palms facing upwards. This is called Bhairavi Mudra, the wrathful form of Parvati the consort of Shiva who kills demons.

Effect: The Palm contains heart related nerve centres and the back of the hand contains the spine related nerve centre. So, placing the palms one upon the other, activate the centres of heart, lings, pancreas and kidneys on one hand and spinal nerve points on the other.

Benefit:

- Dhyana Mudra helps to progress in meditation and the meditator gets pure thoughts and attains peace.
- This Mudra strengthens the muscles in the body. Blood circulation becomes normal.

Mukula Mudra or Samana Mudra

Samana Mudra is also called Mukula Mudra. The formation of this Mudra resembles a bud – Mukula in

Sanskrit. Hence this Mudra is called Mukula Mudra.

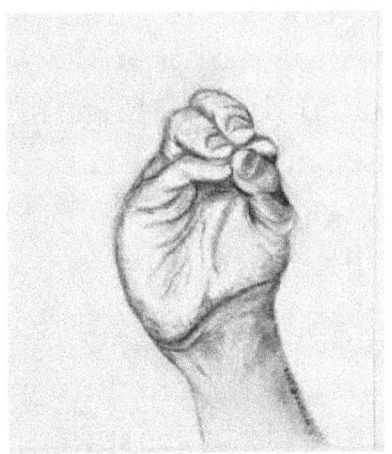

Formation: All the fingers get equal importance with the Agni and they get balanced. This Mudra seems to be simple and is quite effective.

Benefits:

- When this Mudra is placed on the tense or hurting part of the body, it gets relief immediately. It is like directing the energy to a specific part, so one feels instantly rejuvenated. It shaft of the light which is directed to the area of concern. This Mudra is an effective healing tool.

- The electro magnetic forces generated when the five fingers come together is tremendous and that brings about the balance of all elements.

The science of Mudra states that balanced health can be attained if this Mudra is performed at least for 15 minutes a day.

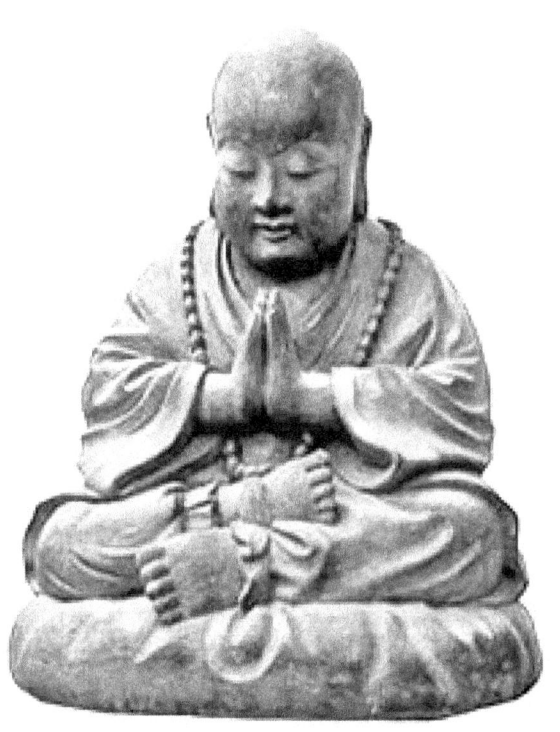

Therapeutic Mudras

Six Mudra are to be practised daily for 10 minutes. They are Jnana, Prithvi, Apana, Dhyana and Vayu – by which disease can be prevented – All should perform these Mudras everyday.

When Mudras are performed for therapy they have to be performed for 50 minutes. One can perform these Mudras several times in a day if time permits. When the disease is controlled then Mudras are to be discontinued. Therapeutic Mudras are followed by Prana Mudra. Persons having the diseases of high blood pressure, cancer or diatese should continue performing the therapeutic Mudras life long.

Linga Mudra is to be performed only for 15 minutes at a time.

A

- Alzimer's problem - Jnana Mudra + Prana Mudra
- Anxiety - Jnana Mudra + Prana Mudra
- Arthritis - Vayu Mudra + Prana Mudra
- Acidity - Surabhi Mudra/ Apana Mudra
- Appetite loss - Surya Mudra
- Anaemia - Prithvi Mudra
- Abdominal pain - Apana Mudra
- Anger - Jnana Mudra
- Acne - Prithvi & Varuna Mudra
- Angina Pectoris - Apana Vayu Mudra

- Asthma   -   Linga + Surya Mudra
- Allergy   - Varuna + Shankha Mudra
- Alertness   -   Jnana Mudra

B

- Blood circulation
  Prana Mudra
- Blood impurity
  Varuna + Prithvi Mudra
- Brittle nails
  Vyana + Prana Mudra
- Backache
  Vayu + Prana Mudra
- Boils
  Varuna + Prana Mudra
- Blocked nose
  Linga Mudra
- Bone pain
  Akasha + Prana Mudra

- Burning urination
  Varuna + Prithvi Mudra

C

- Cervical spondylitis
  Vayu + Samana Mudra
- Creativity
  Surabhi Mudra
- Cerebral Palsy
  Vayu + Prana Mudra
- Cartilage degeneration
  Vayu + Varuna Mudra
- Cancer Eradication
  Gayatri Mudra
- Congestion in the chest
  Linga Mudra
- Cold
  Surya + Linga Mudra

- Cataract
  Surya + Prana Mudra
- Cest pain
  Apana Vayu + Akaash
- Cough wet
  Linga + Surya Mudra
- Cough Dry
  Varuna Mudra

D

- Dehydration
  Varuna Mudra
- Depression
  Mushthi + Prana Mudra
- Diabetes   Apana
  + Prana Mudra

- Diarrhea
  Jalodara Nashak Mudra
- Dry mouth
  Varuna Mudra
- Dixxiness
  Shoonya Mudra
- Digestion problem   Surya
  + Linga Mudra

E

- Ear ache
  Akasha + Shoonya Mudra
- Egoism
  Jnana Mudra
- Emotional Imbalance
  Surabhi + Jnana Mudra
- Energy
  Surya + Prana Mudra

- Exhaustion
  Prana + Prithvi Mudra
- Excess Sweating,

  Drowsiness
  Vyana Mudra

F

- Fatigue
  Prana + Surya Mudra
- Fear
  Jnana + Prana Mudra
- For painless delivery
  Apana Mudra
- Fever
  Prithvi Mudra
- Fits - Vayu + Varuna+ Prana
- Fever due to cold
  Surya + Pankaja Mudra

G

- Gastroenteritis
  Varuna Mudra

H

- Headache –
  Apana Vayu + Prana Mudra
- Heart problem
  Akash + Apana + Prana Mudra
- Heartbeat skipping
  Apana Vayu Mudra
- Hiccups
  Apana Vayu Mudra
- Heart problem
  Apana + Prana Mudra

I

- Immunity to develop
  Prana Mudra
- Insomnia
  Jnana + Prana Mudra
- Intution Power
  Akash + Jnana Mudra
- Irritation
  Jnana Mudra
- Itching
  Varuna Mudra

J

- Jalodar
  Jalodhar Nashak Mudra
- Jaundice
  Prithvi + Prana Mudra
- Jet Lag prevention
  Akasha + Prana Mudra

K

- Kidney problem
  Apana / Apana Vayu/ Jala
- Knee pain
  Vayu + Varuna + Prana Mudra
- Knowledge
  Jnana Mudra

L

- Laziness
  Jnana + Prithvi + Prana Mudra
- Liver problem
  Surya + Shankha + sahaja
  Mudra

M

- Meditation
  Jnana + Dhyana + Akasha
  Mudra
- Memory power
  Jnana + Prana Mudra
- Mental problem
  Jnana + Prana Mudra
- Migraine
  Apana Vayu + Prana Mudra
- Muscle catch
  Vayu + Varuna + Prana Mudra

N

- Navel disorder
  Shankha/ Linga Mudra
- Neck ache
  Vayu + Namaskara Mudra

O

- Obesity
  Surya + Linga Mudra
- Obsession
  Jnana Mudra
- Obstinacy
  Jnana Mudra + Prana Mudra
- Over Urination
  Jalodara Nashaka Mudra

P

- Paralysis
  Vayu + Prana Mudra
- Parkinson disease
  Vayu + Prana + Jnana Mudra
- Periods problem
  Yoni Mudra

- Piles
  Sahaja Shankha Mudra
- Pitta
  Surabhi Mudra
- Pieurisy
  Linga + Prana Mudra
- Polio
  Vayu + Prana + Prithvi Mudra
- Purification of nerves
  Prana + Shankha Mudra

R

- Restlessness
  Jnana Mudra
- Rudeness
  Jnana + Pankaja Mudra

S

- Sinus
  Linga + Surya Mudra
- Skin problem
  Varuna + Apana Mudra
- Sneezing cont...
  Aditi Mudra
- Stammering
  Sahaja + Jnana Mudra
- Stiff Jaw
  Akash Mudra
- Swelling
  Jalodar Nashak Mudra
- Sciatica
  Vayu + Prana Mudra

T

- Teeth problem
  Akash + Apana Mudra

- Tension
  Jnana Mudra
- Thirst
  Varuna + Prana Mudra
- Tonsillitis
  Shankha Mudra
- Tuberculosis
  Linga + Suya Mudra

U

- Unconsciousness
  Varuna Mudra to be rubbed.

V

- Vayu disorder
  Vayu Mudra
- Vomiting
  Apan + Apana Vayu Mudra

- Vital energy
  Prana Mudra

W

- Weakness
  Prithvi + Prana Mudra
- Weight gain
  Aditi Mudra
- Wish fulfilling
  Surabhi Mudra

Y

- Yawning
  Aditi Mudra

Use Mudra for healing yourself, your soul with

Voice Print Mudra program

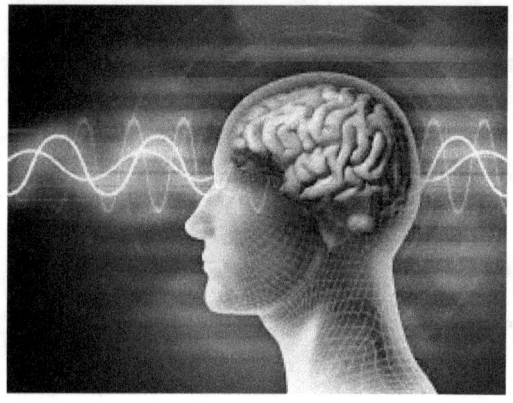

Yoga and Health

Yoga is the ancient cultural heritage of India. It is a great contribution to the world community in the venture of cultivating humanity at its best.

The term Yoga is derived from the Sanskrit root Yuji to unite the human consciousness with the divine consciousness.

Mahashi Patanjali's name is identified with Yoga as he gathered together and codified the principles that were scattered in many philosophical texts.

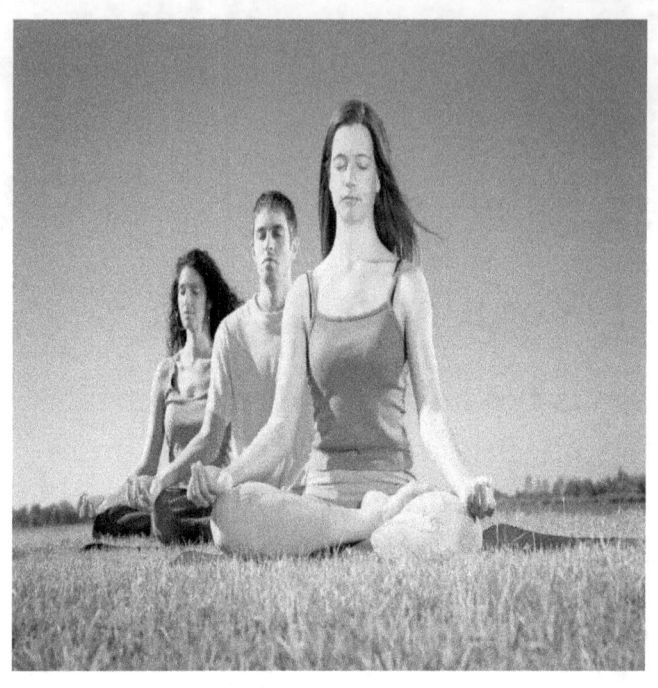

Yoga Sutra of Patanjali dates back to around 300 B.C. It is an integrated system as it addresses to both man's gross body and subtle body on physical, mental and intellectual levels.

Maharshi Patanjali's work is in the form of Sutras or short Aphorism.

This work is primarily a practical and to develop a brilliant intuitive mind that brings about spiritual realization.

Yoga has universal application, can be tried by any adult follower of any religion or region.

There are mainly four streams of yoga.

1. Jnana Yoga - gaining Knowledge by contemplation.
2. Raja Yoga - Phychic control and culturing the mind.
3. Karma Yoga – Incentive oriented work.
4. Bhakti Yoga – Culturing of emotions.

Through Yoga practice – One progresses from darkness to light, weakness to strength diversity to unity and ignorance to enlightenment.

Yoga is a message of Peace.

The Philosophy of Life & health:

The body and mind are inseparable. They are like the two sides of a coin. The coin gets out of mode even when one side is worn out. Similarly health of the body and mind is closely interralated.

From ancient times it is a tradition in India to emphasise and seek internal happiness than the external show. The contemplative often asked the challenging questions "Who am I?" and the prompt answer was "I am Atma – the Soul.

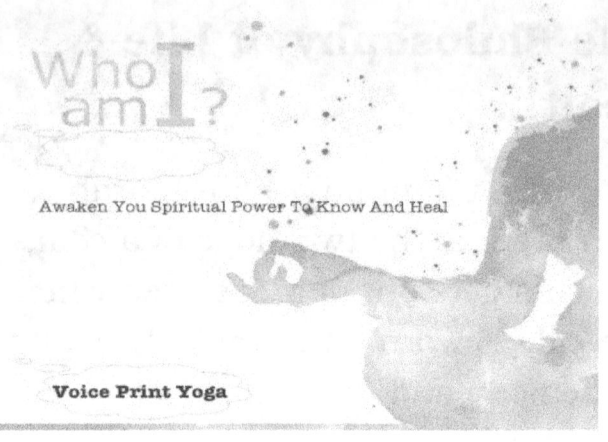

" I am Atma – the Soul"

Spirit is soul, immaterial, intellectual or moral part of man. Spirituality captures the spirit of philosophy, ethics and values. It is not a ritualistic religious activity but promotes certain commonly universal values, creates balance in need and greed.

There are six enemies of the spirit that lead to the distruction of man. They are

   1. Kama   passion
   2. Krodha   anger
   3. Lobha   greed
   4. Moha   infatuation
   5. Mada   pride
   6. Matsarya   Jealousy

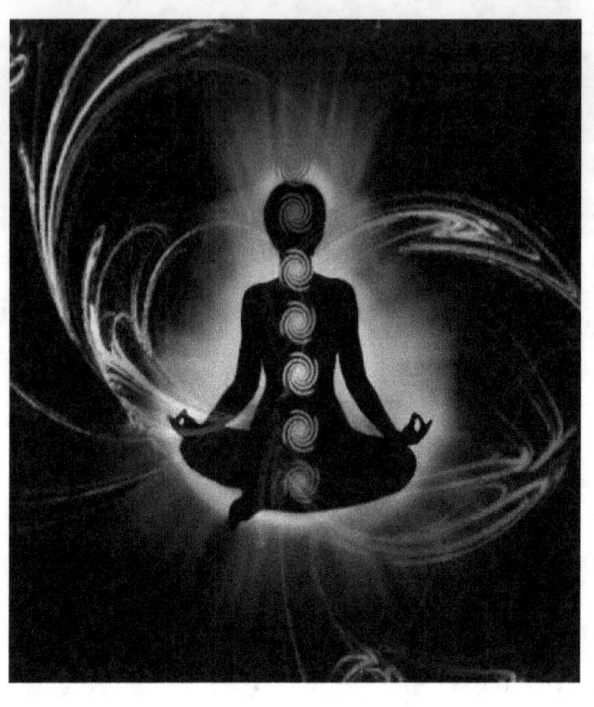

Organs that are affected with negative emotions are as following

Emotions
Organs

- *Anxiety & sense adrenals*
  Of lack of support
- *Insecurity*
  bladder
- *Sense of lack of love*
  heart
- *Sadness and grief*
  lungs
- *Fear*
  kidney
- *Hate*
  gall bladder
- *Anger*
  liver
- *Fear of failure*
  small intestine

- *Greed, attachment,*
  Possessiveness
  spleen
- *Lack of fulfilment*
  stomach

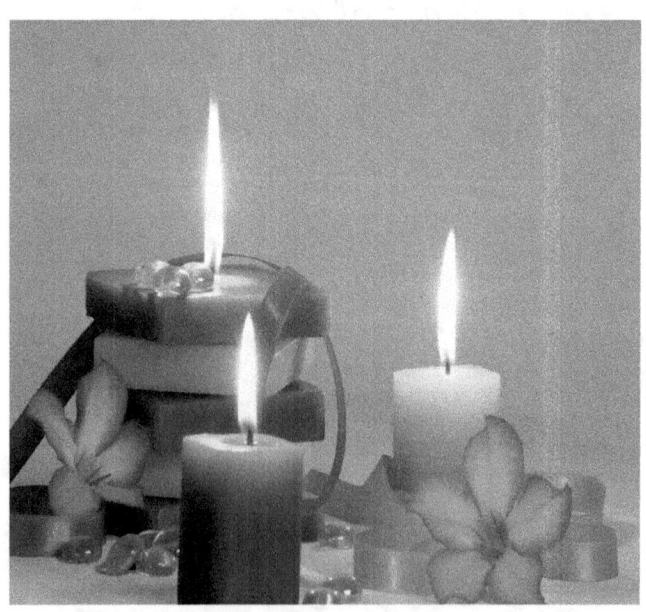

The Significance of Mantra:

Mantra refers to a divine name or a spiritual mystic formula which is repeated with devotion and understanding for attaining material prosperity, health and spiritual illumination.

Japa is the repetition of a mantra orally or mentally.

Mala is a rosary of 108 beads which help the repetition of mantra.

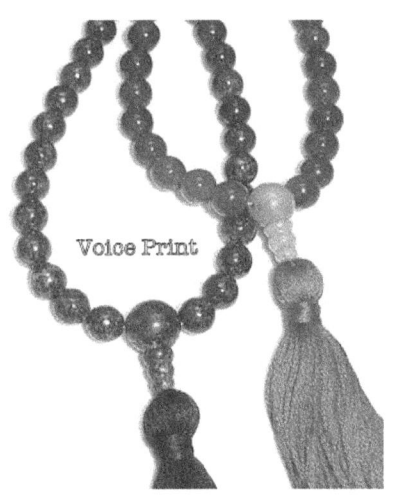

Heart is the seat of Atma and from the heart spring 108 nerves (nadis) which send the vibrations through out the body. So it is interesting to note that the minimum number of Mantras to be chanted is 108 times which would activate the nerves of the heart.

Mantra may consist of a brief prayer, the name or an aspect of the divinity, or a collection of Sanskrit root letters – the Beejaksharas.

Mantra consists of letter or words well calculated to bring about specific results by awakening psychic power. Mantra is the key to unlock a potential treasure within.

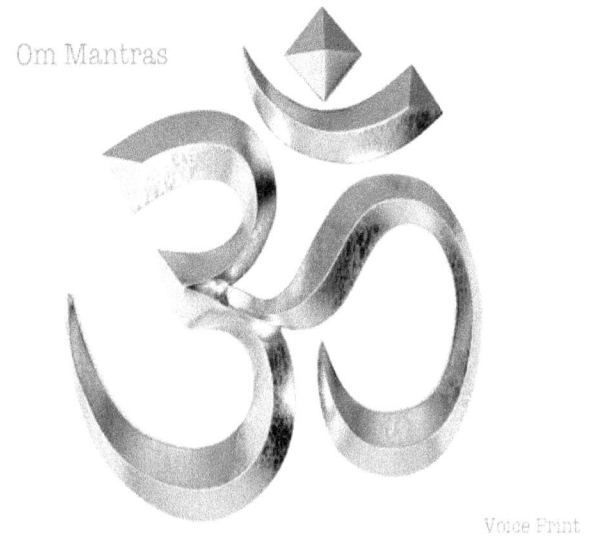

Voice print Om mantra chanting

OM is the mother of all the Mantras, it is the source of all words and sounds.

Therefore OM describes the most perfect symbol or name of the supreme.

When Mantra is chanted, gradually the mind assumes a state of purity and serenity.

In this ascending movement of mental purification, concentration and meditation, the higher thought waves which were obstructed before, now begin to manifest enriching one's life with insight and spiritual strength.

OM is the sound which projected the universe. During the cosmic dissolution the universe merged in OM.

OM is beyond time, space and causation. All Vedic Mantra have emerged from OM and begin with OM.

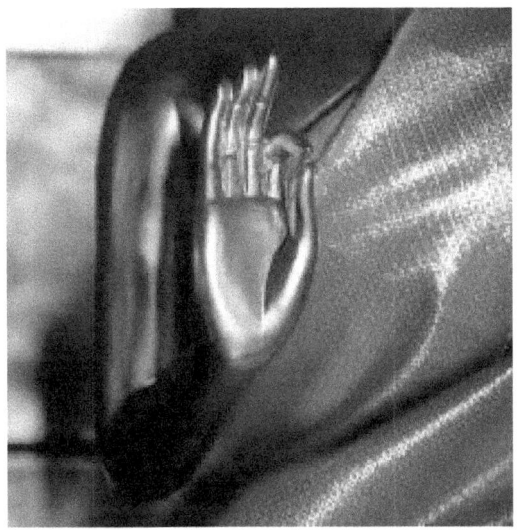

Voice Print Yoga

Voice Print Yoga is specially designed by my experience through travelling and my stay in Himalayas.

Voice Print is a yoga of vibration healing, vibration energising. Voice Print Yoga along with practise of Mudras & Mantras will open your Chakras and develop your mind towards *Moksha*.

The Earth Vibrations are a basis for healing.
With modern society bombarding us with so much electromagnetic energy, it seems increasingly obvious that getting more in tune with the Earth energy is universally healing. People who leave big, noisy cities and move out to the country enjoy spectacular health improvements. People who contact the earth through gardening,

outdoors activities or consuming natural foods are far healthier than those who don't. And almost everyone agrees that a lush, green forest, humming with life, is calming and healing to both the mind and body.

If you want to help people, your loved one and this planet just get is touch with the frequency of earth, the obvious thing to do is get them vibrating at multiples of the earth frequency.

Voice Print yoga is a science to increase your vibrations.

Vibrational medicine is one of the most, if not the most widely studied field of medicine today. There is now global interest and research in the clinical applications of Vibrational Medicine.

Mudras can help you to balance your body elements.

Voice Print De-stress

program

The Gayatri Mantra

Om Bhoor Bhuvah Svah
Tat Savitur Varenyam
Bhargo Devasya Dheemahi
Dhiyo Yonah Prachodayaat.

ॐ भूर्भुवः स्वः
तत्सवितुर्वरेण्यं
भर्गो देवस्य धीमहि
धियो योनः प्रचोदयात् ।

Oh Creator of the Universe!
We meditate upon thy supreme splendor.
May thy radiant power illuminate our intellects,
destroy our sins, and guide us in the right direction!

New Releases By Yoga Karma:

Books

- **Yoga Soul & Vibration**
- **Mudras**

Music

- **OM Mantra (108 Om chanting)**
- *Voice Print* **Meditation Music**
- *Voice Print* **Trans Meditation Music**

Coming soon:

- **Who am I ?**
- **Aakashic Records**

We are travellers; this life is our stopover...

Yogi Karma

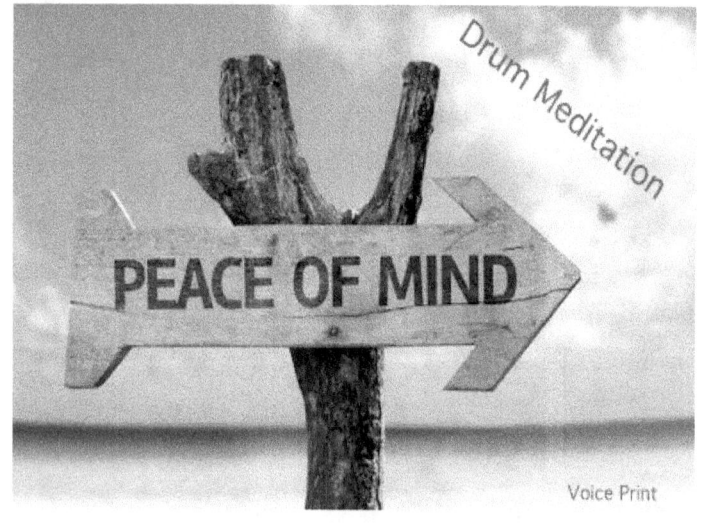

Drum Meditation

PEACE OF MIND

Voice Print

www.ingramcontent.com/pod-product-compliance
Lightning Source LLC
Chambersburg PA
CBHW070655290526
45790CB00001B/332